SECRET HERBAL REMEDIES OF THE EDUCATORS

Secret Herbal Remedies of the Educators

Walter the Educator

Silent King Books

SILENT KING BOOKS

SKB

Copyright © 2024 by Walter the Educator

All rights reserved. No part of this book may be reproduced in any manner whatsoever without written permission except in the case of brief quotations embodied in critical articles and reviews.

First Printing, 2024

Disclaimer
This book is a literary work; poems are not about specific persons, locations, situations, and/or circumstances unless mentioned in a historical context. This book is for entertainment and informational purposes only. The author and publisher offer this information without warranties expressed or implied. No matter the grounds, neither the author nor the publisher will be accountable for any losses, injuries, or other damages caused by the reader's use of this book. The use of this book acknowledges an understanding and acceptance of this disclaimer.

dedicated to those that love collecting little books

SECRET HERBAL REMEDIES OF THE EDUCATORS

Aloe Vera: Known for its soothing and anti-inflammatory properties, aloe vera is excellent for treating burns, cuts, and skin irritations. It also aids in digestion and can help alleviate constipation.

**Secret
Herbal Remedies
of the
Educators**

Chamomile: This calming herb is often used to promote relaxation and sleep. Chamomile tea can help soothe digestive issues, reduce menstrual pain, and alleviate stress.

Secret
Herbal Remedies
of the
Educators

Echinacea: Commonly used to boost the immune system, echinacea can help prevent and treat colds, flu, and other infections. It also has anti-inflammatory and antioxidant properties.

**Secret
Herbal Remedies
of the
Educators**

Lavender: Known for its calming and relaxing effects, lavender can help reduce anxiety, improve sleep, and relieve headaches. It's also useful in treating minor burns and insect bites.

**Secret
Herbal Remedies
of the
Educators**

Peppermint: This herb is great for relieving digestive issues such as bloating, gas, and indigestion. Peppermint oil can also alleviate headaches and muscle pain.

**Secret
Herbal Remedies
of the
Educators**

Ginger: Widely used for its anti-nausea and anti-inflammatory properties, ginger is effective in treating motion sickness, morning sickness, and digestive problems. It also helps reduce muscle pain and soreness.

Secret
Herbal Remedies
of the
Educators

Turmeric: Rich in curcumin, turmeric has powerful anti-inflammatory and antioxidant properties. It's beneficial for joint health, reducing inflammation, and improving liver function.

**Secret
Herbal Remedies
of the
Educators**

St. John's Wort: Often used to treat mild to moderate depression and anxiety, St. John's Wort also has antiviral and anti-inflammatory properties. It can help with wound healing and nerve pain.

Secret
Herbal Remedies
of the
Educators

Garlic: Known for its immune-boosting properties, garlic helps fight infections, lower blood pressure, and improve cardiovascular health. It also has anti-inflammatory and antioxidant benefits.

**Secret
Herbal Remedies
of the
Educators**

Rosemary: This herb enhances memory and concentration. Rosemary oil is useful for relieving muscle pain and improving hair growth. It also has antimicrobial properties.

Secret
Herbal Remedies
of the
Educators

Sage: Used to improve memory and brain function, sage also helps with digestive issues and sore throats. It has antimicrobial and anti-inflammatory properties.

**Secret
Herbal Remedies
of the
Educators**

Thyme: Rich in antioxidants, thyme is great for boosting the immune system and treating respiratory conditions like bronchitis and coughs. It also has antimicrobial properties.

Secret
Herbal Remedies
of the
Educators

Lemon Balm: Known for its calming effects, lemon balm helps reduce anxiety, improve sleep, and alleviate digestive issues. It's also effective in treating cold sores.

Secret
Herbal Remedies
of the
Educators

Milk Thistle: Primarily used to support liver health, milk thistle helps detoxify the liver, reduce inflammation, and improve skin health.

Secret
Herbal Remedies
of the
Educators

Dandelion: This herb is a natural diuretic and supports liver health. Dandelion also aids in digestion and helps with skin conditions like acne.

**Secret
Herbal Remedies
of the
Educators**

Calendula: Known for its healing properties, calendula is excellent for treating skin conditions, wounds, and burns. It also has anti-inflammatory and antimicrobial benefits.

**Secret
Herbal Remedies
of the
Educators**

Elderberry: Commonly used to boost the immune system, elderberry helps treat colds, flu, and respiratory infections. It also has antioxidant and anti-inflammatory properties.

**Secret
Herbal Remedies
of the
Educators**

Valerian Root: Effective in promoting relaxation and improving sleep, valerian root helps reduce anxiety and muscle spasms.

**Secret
Herbal Remedies
of the
Educators**

Ashwagandha: This adaptogenic herb helps reduce stress, improve cognitive function, and boost energy levels. It also supports immune health and hormonal balance.

**Secret
Herbal Remedies
of the
Educators**

Holy Basil: Known for its adaptogenic properties, holy basil helps reduce stress, improve respiratory function, and support immune health.

**Secret
Herbal Remedies
of the
Educators**

Fenugreek: Often used to improve digestion, fenugreek also helps lower blood sugar levels, reduce inflammation, and enhance milk production in breastfeeding mothers.

**Secret
Herbal Remedies
of the
Educators**

Hawthorn: Beneficial for heart health, hawthorn helps improve circulation, reduce blood pressure, and alleviate chest pain. It also has antioxidant properties.

**Secret
Herbal Remedies
of the
Educators**

Nettle: Known for its anti-inflammatory and detoxifying properties, nettle helps treat allergies, support joint health, and improve skin conditions.

**Secret
Herbal Remedies
of the
Educators**

Ginseng: This adaptogen boosts energy levels, improves cognitive function, and supports immune health. It also helps reduce stress and enhance physical performance.

Secret
Herbal Remedies
of the
Educators

Bilberry: Rich in antioxidants, bilberry helps improve vision, support cardiovascular health, and reduce inflammation.

**Secret
Herbal Remedies
of the
Educators**

Cinnamon: Known for its blood sugar-regulating properties, cinnamon helps improve digestion, reduce inflammation, and boost immune health.

**Secret
Herbal Remedies
of the
Educators**

Licorice Root: This herb helps soothe the digestive tract, reduce inflammation, and improve respiratory health. It's also effective in treating adrenal fatigue.

**Secret
Herbal Remedies
of the
Educators**

Burdock Root: Used for detoxifying the liver and blood, burdock root helps improve skin health, support digestion, and reduce inflammation.

**Secret
Herbal Remedies
of the
Educators**

Goldenseal: Known for its antimicrobial and immune-boosting properties, goldenseal helps treat infections, support digestive health, and reduce inflammation.

**Secret
Herbal Remedies
of the
Educators**

Passionflower: Effective in promoting relaxation and reducing anxiety, passionflower also helps improve sleep and alleviate pain.

Secret
Herbal Remedies
of the
Educators

Yarrow: This herb helps reduce inflammation, improve digestion, and promote wound healing. It also has antimicrobial properties.

**Secret
Herbal Remedies
of the
Educators**

Catnip: Known for its calming effects, catnip helps reduce anxiety, improve sleep, and alleviate digestive issues.

**Secret
Herbal Remedies
of the
Educators**

Mullein: Used to treat respiratory conditions, mullein helps reduce inflammation, soothe the throat, and improve lung health.

**Secret
Herbal Remedies
of the
Educators**

Red Clover: This herb supports hormonal balance, improves skin health, and reduces inflammation. It's also used to support cardiovascular health.

Secret
Herbal Remedies
of the
Educators

Slippery Elm: Known for its soothing effects on the digestive tract, slippery elm helps treat ulcers, acid reflux, and sore throats.

**Secret
Herbal Remedies
of the
Educators**

Basil: This herb helps reduce inflammation, improve digestion, and support immune health. It also has antimicrobial properties.

**Secret
Herbal Remedies
of the
Educators**

Oregano: Rich in antioxidants, oregano helps boost the immune system, improve digestion, and treat respiratory conditions. It also has antimicrobial properties.

Secret
Herbal Remedies
of the
Educators

Marshmallow Root: Used for its soothing effects on the digestive and respiratory tracts, marshmallow root helps treat coughs, colds, and digestive issues.

**Secret
Herbal Remedies
of the
Educators**

Comfrey: Known for its healing properties, comfrey helps treat wounds, sprains, and fractures. It also reduces inflammation and supports skin health.

**Secret
Herbal Remedies
of the
Educators**

Motherwort: This herb is often used to support heart health, reduce anxiety, and alleviate menstrual pain. It also has anti-inflammatory and antimicrobial properties.

**Secret
Herbal Remedies
of the
Educators**

ABOUT THE CREATOR

Walter the Educator is one of the pseudonyms for Walter Anderson. Formally educated in Chemistry, Business, and Education, he is an educator, an author, a diverse entrepreneur, and he is the son of a disabled war veteran. "Walter the Educator" shares his time between educating and creating. He holds interests and owns several creative projects that entertain, enlighten, enhance, and educate, hoping to inspire and motivate you.

Follow, find new works, and stay up to date
with Walter the Educator™
at WaltertheEducator.com

www.ingramcontent.com/pod-product-compliance
Lightning Source LLC
LaVergne TN
LVHW010412070526
838199LV00064B/5270